# FIX YOUR GUT

## And Get Relief from Celiac, Crohn's, IBD, IBS, GERD, and more

Terri Eileen Liggins

The Literary Front Publishing Company
Las Vegas, Nevada, USA

Published by The Literary Front Publishing Company
Las Vegas, Nevada, U.S.A.

ISBN 978-1-7366866-2-1

# Dedication

I dedicate this book to anyone who has dealt with or is currently dealing with digestive problems of any kind. If you suffer from celiac, GERD, inflammatory bowel disease, such as ulcerative colitis and Crohn's disease, irritable bowel syndrome, gallstones, iron deficiency and many other sicknesses, just know relief is at your fingertips. Just flip the pages of this book.

I love and care about you and your well-being. So, right now sit back, relax, take a deep breath, read this book in its entirety, and know that your healing is waiting on you.

## Acknowledgments

Every day, I wake up thanking God for another opportunity to fulfill my purpose. And to do so in prosperous health, just as my soul prospers.

I acknowledge with gratitude my loved ones, whether family, friends or colleagues, who show up for me—believing in me, cheering me on, holding me accountable, praying for me, purchasing from me, and just letting me be me. Thank you all.

# I Deliver Value, Then They Say These Sweet Things...

"You are a master, and I appreciate you more than I can express.

~ *Monalisa Jones*

"Greatly appreciate all that you are doing!!! ...Your work is invaluable. I have overcome many health issues because of you & your alliances. Thanks for the feedback so that I can move forward in using your services. God Bless!!!!"

~ *Wanda White*

"I believe Terri has the ability to empower and encourage her readers to create the best version of themselves—whether she's talking health matters or helping someone write their book. I am forever grateful for her professional and expert ability to make editorial adjustments in persona, tone, and voice to transform the oral history of my 32-year political career into my written living memoir. I highly recommend that you connect with her."

~ *Roland Burris II, Retired U.S. Senator (IL-D)*

"This book is for anyone who wants to get ahead of the health game… It's the perfect set-it-and-forget-it guide you didn't know you needed."
~ *Skye Shepard, Actress*

"You always are an inspiration to me Auntie… I love your spirit, your wisdom, your energy, and your willingness to always have your mind open to learn more!! You have set the standard very high and I LOVE YOU for THAT!
~ *John Harris III*

"Terri Liggins is an empowering, inspiring and motivating woman on a mission to help you THRIVE. Her own evolutionary journey has infused her with the knowledge and wisdom to support you in elevating your physical, mental and emotion wellbeing. I highly recommend allowing Terri to support you step by step toward your best self and best life."
~ *Chara Rodriguera, Inspirational Yoga Teacher, Author and Facilitator at Chara.tv.*

"Terri - My tenacious, ever Ready and Real Integrity Friend. She has been able to reach, with such grace, respect and dedication to helping others achieve their goals. Her book is a perfect example of her willingness to care about others."

*~ Cheryl Martin, Vocalist, Owner at Integrity Bookkeeping Services*

"So excited for you!! You inspire me, friend!"

~ Kim Watt, Owner Bruster's Ice Cream, Matthews, NC

"Terri, thank you for sharing and caring about our health. When we know better, we should do better."

*~ Pam Jackson*

"I had no idea that there is more than being a vegetarian. Rawtarian is something that is out of my radar but let me tell you that the context of this book is really intelligent, and I believe it is something that people should be knowledgeable about... That is why I believe this book should reach more people. Very informative and empathetic."

*~ Mae Diestro, Breastfeeding Mom*

"Your posts are so informative, thank you!"

*~ Senetta Barton- Almira*

"Terri Eileen Liggins, you are consistently giving us

#HealthGoals! THANK YOU for all of this information! I appreciate it and you."
~ *Sherma Jacqueline Felix, CEO/Founder, The Black Advantage Group, LLC*

"It was truly wonderful and informative. You have a great presence, Terri, and we all learn so much from you."
~ *Mary Hida*

"You were born to inspire, inform, and excite. Keep on learning and doing that which is right."
~ *Chef Keidi Awadu, Founder, Living Superfood*

"Gotta love you, Terri Eileen Liggins. You are definitely RAW funny and down to EARTH for real."
~ *Lindy Irving*

"Everything you post is so amazing looking! And healthy!"
~ *Debbie King*

"Cousin, I love your platform. You inspire me so much!"
~ *Erin Liggins @TheWriterErin*

"Please keep inspiring. Your light shines bright!"
~ *Tiffany Mayes Eholor, Owner, Tribal Exchange*

"I can't thank you enough. You are making an impact in so many ways. You're my Shero! Stay Blessed."
~ *Michael J. Roebuck*

# Disclaimer

**Before you enjoy this publication, please take heed to my disclaimer.**

All the material written in this document is provided for informational purposes only and is general in nature.

Every person is a unique individual and what has worked for some, or even many, may not work for you. Any information perceived as advice must be considered in light of your own set of circumstances.

The author or person sharing this information does not assume any responsibility for the accuracy or outcome of your use of the content.

Every attempt has been made to provide well-researched and up-to-date content at the time of writing. Nevertheless, you should consult a healthcare provider, nutritionist or other qualified professional for your own diagnosis and consultation before making any changes to your diet and/or exercise routine. Also, you should never stop taking medication without first consulting the physician who prescribed it.

Now that all the legalities have been taken care of, happy reading to you!

# Table of Contents

# Chapter 1:
# What Is Your Digestive System?

We hear about, read about, or talk about our digestive system all the time but do we really know what it is? What organs comprise the digestive system? What is the true function of it? Most importantly, how can we protect it so that it helps deliver longevity in return?

The Digestive System

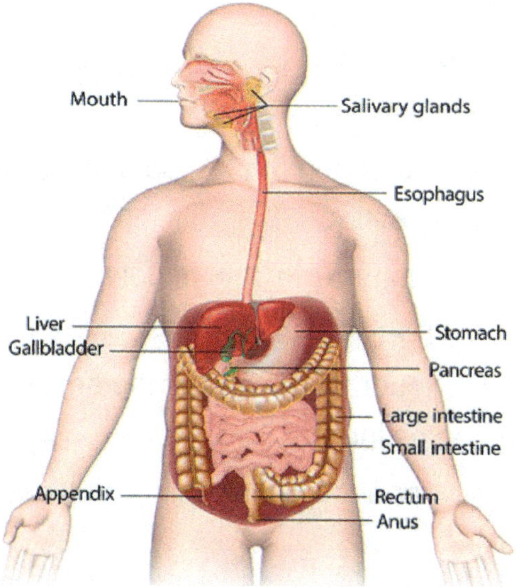

The digestive system is made up of the gastrointestinal tract (the GI tract or digestive tract), and the liver, pancreas, and gallbladder. The GI tract is a series of hollow organs joined in a long, twisting tube that extends from the mouth to the anus. The liver, pancreas and gallbladder are the solid organs of.

**Here is an outline of those hollow and solid organs**

The six hollow organs

- mouth
- esophagus
- stomach
- small intestine
  - duodenum, in the beginning of the small intestine
  - jejunum, in the middle of the small intestine
  - ileum, at the end of the small intestine
- large intestine
  - appendix, a finger-shaped pouch

attached to the cecum

    - cecum, at the beginning of the large intestine
    - colon, goes from the small intestine to the rectum
    - rectum, at the lower end of the large intestine

- anus

The three solid organs

- liver,
- pancreas
- gallbladder

# Chapter 2: How Does The Digestive Process Work?

Food moves through your GI tract via a process called peristalsis. The large, hollow organs of your GI tract contain a layer of muscle that enables their walls to move through your GI tract and mixes the food contents inside each of the organs. These muscles are contracts and squeezes the food forward, while the muscle in front of the food relaxes to allow the food to advance through without incident.

Each part of your digestive system helps to move food and liquid through your GI tract, break food and liquid into smaller parts, or both. Once foods are broken into small enough parts, your body can absorb and move the nutrients to where they are needed. Your large intestine absorbs water, and the waste products of digestion become stool. Nerves and hormones help control the digestive process.

**The six hollow organs**

**Mouth.** Food starts to move through your GI tract when you eat. When you swallow, your tongue pushes the food into your throat. A small flap of tissue, called the epiglottis, folds over your windpipe to prevent choking and the food passes into your esophagus.

**Esophagus.** Once you begin swallowing, the process becomes automatic. Your brain signals the muscles of the esophagus and peristalsis begins. When food reaches the end of your esophagus, a ringlike muscle—called the lower esophageal sphincter —relaxes and lets food pass into your stomach. This sphincter usually stays closed to keep what's in your stomach from flowing back into your esophagus.

**Stomach.** After food enters your stomach, the stomach muscles mix the food and liquid with digestive juices. The stomach slowly empties its contents, called chyme, into your small intestine.

**Small intestine.** The muscles of the small intestine mix food with more digestive juices; this time from the pancreas, liver, and intestine. That mixture is then pushed forward for further digestion. The walls of the small intestine absorb water and the digested nutrients into your bloodstream. As peristalsis continues, the waste products of the digestive process move into the large intestine.

<u>Here are the organs that make up the small intestine</u>:

The **duodenum** is a vital part of the digestive system. It is a tubular structure that starts at the stomach and connects to the small intestine and is only 10 inches (typically the length of the webbing between the thumb and forefinger). The duodenum plays an important role in digesting food and absorbing nutrients. When you eat, food enters the stomach and is mixed with stomach acids. These acids break down the food, making it easier for the body to absorb nutrients. The duodenum helps to further break down the food while absorbing some nutrients itself. Without a functioning duodenum, we would not be able to properly digest our food or absorb the nutrients we need to survive.

The **jejunum** is the middle section of the small intestine and measures about 2 feet long. It is where most of the nutrient absorption takes place in the gastrointestinal tract. It extends from the duodenum (the first section of the small intestine) to the ileum (the last section of the small intestine). The jejunum is characterized by its large surface area, which is due to its many folds of mucosa. This large surface area allows for a greater absorption of nutrients from food. The jejunum also has a higher concentration of enzymes than the other sections of the small intestine, which aids in digestion.

The **ileum** is the last part of the small intestine. It is about 2 to 3 feet long. It begins at the jejunum and ends at the large intestine (colon). The ileum absorbs most of the nutrients from food. It contains lymphatic nodules, which are masses of lymphatic tissue that produce white blood cells to fight infection. The wall of the ileum also has numerous Peyer's patches, which are collections of lymphoid tissue. These patches help protect against infection by trapping bacteria and other foreign particles in the intestinal lumen.

**Large intestine.** Waste products from the digestive process include undigested parts of food, fluid, and older cells from the lining of your GI tract. The large intestine absorbs water and changes the waste from liquid into stool. Peristalsis helps move the stool into your rectum.

<u>Here are the organs that make up the large intestine</u>:

The **appendix** is a small, tube-shaped organ that hangs down from the large intestine. It is 2 to 4 inches and shaped like a finger. The appendix really has no known function. Some experts think the appendix may help with digestion, but there's no evidence that it does. Others think it helps fight infection, but again, there's no evidence to support this claim. Most people don't need their appendix removed, but if it becomes infected or swollen, it can be dangerous, so surgery to remove the appendix is often recommended.

The **cecum** is a pouch that is located at the beginning of the large intestine. The small intestine empties into the cecum, which is where digestion of food takes place. Some of the contents of the cecum include undigested food, bacteria, and mucus. The primary function of the cecum is to hold these substances until they can be passed on to the rest of the intestines for further digestion or elimination from the body. There are a few other functions of the cecum as well. For example, it aids in water absorption and electrolyte balance, and it also produces some vitamins (such as K) that are essential for good health.

The **colon** is a coiled section of the large intestine that runs from the small intestine to the rectum. It is about 5 feet long and is where most of the water is reabsorbed from fecal matter before it exits the body as feces. The colon is also responsible for extracting nutrients and minerals from food before that food is eliminated from the body as solid waste (stool) through the rectum during a bowel movement.

The **rectum** is the final section and lower end of the

large intestine, connecting the colon to the anus. It is about 4.7 inches long, and is divided into three sections: the upper, middle, and lower rectum. The word “rectum” comes from the Latin rectus meaning “straight.” It stores feces (stool) until it pushes the stool out of the anus during a bowel movement. When feces enter there, they stimulate nerves in the rectum, which send signals to the brain telling you it’s time to have a bowel movement. Isn’t it simply miraculous how the body operates?

**Anus.** The anus is the rectal opening through which feces is excreted. It is located at the end of the gastrointestinal tract and typically considered to be a dirty and taboo subject. However, it plays such an important role in keeping our digestive system functioning properly that no one should shy away from discussions about it. Another description of the anus is a muscular ring as the terminal opening of the alimentary canal. The alimentary canal is a long tube that runs from the mouth to the anus (which explains the slang “from the rooter to the tooter”). The alimentary canal includes the esophagus, stomach, small intestine, and large intestine.

**The three solid organs**

**Liver.** During the digesting process, as our food is breaking down, nutrients are being absorbed into the bloodstream. The liver's vital role encompasses many functions. For instance, it filters harmful substances from getting into the bloodstream, helps to regulate metabolism, produces bile which is essential in breaking down fats, stores nutrients and energy, and synthesizes essential proteins. It also aids in metabolizing carbohydrates, fats, and proteins.

Whew! What *doesn't* the liver do? If this doesn't convince you how important it is for you to take care of your liver, I don't know what would. Simply put, without a healthy liver, your body cannot function properly.

**Pancreas.** The pancreas is an exocrine gland that produces digestive enzymes. These enzymes help break down food in the small intestine. The pancreas is also an endocrine gland that produces hormones, such as insulin and glucagon. The hormones help to regulate blood sugar levels and energy metabolism. Insulin helps to keep blood sugar levels stable by causing cells to take up glucose from the bloodstream, while glucagon helps to increase blood sugar levels by causing the liver to release stored glucose.

The pancreas is located behind the stomach and has two parts: the head (which is closest to the stomach) and the tail (which is closest to the small intestine). The head of the pancreas contains clusters of cells called acini, which produce digestive enzymes. The tail of the pancreas contains clusters of cells called ducts, which secrete insulin and other hormones into the bloodstream.

**Gallbladder.** The gallbladder is a small pear-shaped organ that lies on the right side of the abdomen. It stores and concentrates bile containing cholesterol, bilirubin, and other things, which is used to digest fat and remove toxins from the blood. Bile is made in the liver and released into small ducts that merge to form the larger common bile duct. The common bile duct empties into the duodenum (first part of the small intestine), just past the stomach.

Sometimes, the liver doesn't produce enough bile, or the duct that carries bile from the liver to the small intestine gets blocked. When this happens, the gallbladder can also release bile directly into the small intestine. This is called "cholecystokinin-pancreozymin secretion."

# Good Nutrition

# =

# Good Digestion

*Good nutrition is really not rocket science. Good nutrition is all about eating the right foods in the right amounts. It's not aboutperfect eating or following a strict diet – it's about making small, sustainable changes that will make a big impact on your overall health.*

*Three key components to good nutrition are:1) Eating a variety of nutrient-rich foods.2) Consuming theright amount of calories for your individual needs. 3) Making sure those calories come from healthy, balanced sources.*

# Chapter 3: Friendly Bacteria In Digestive Health

Most people do not realize our gut is filled with bacteria all the time. Most of the bacteria and fungi in our system exist in the colon. In fact, it is estimated that, at any given point in time, several pounds of bacteria exist in our system.

Bacteria in your GI tract, also called gut flora or microbiome, help with digestion. Parts of your nervous and circulatory systems help as well. Your nerves, hormones, bacteria, blood, and the organs of your digestive system all work together to digest the foods and liquids you eat or drink each day.

**Friendly Bacteria versus Unfriendly Bacteria**

If our digestive system is working properly, it consists

mostly of friendly bacteria. These consist of bacteria that come from the Bifidobacterium family, Acidophilus, and Lactobacillus family of bacteria. There are about 100 trillion of these bacteria that actually outnumber the number of cells in the actual human body by a factor of 10:1.

Friendly bacteria live in a symbiotic relationship with us. They aid in the proper metabolism of nutrients we eat. Some nutrients we consume cannot be utilized by the body until they are first metabolized by the friendly bacteria. The bacteria use the nutrients we provide for them in the gut and use them for fuel, exchanging them for nutrients our body needs. Without the help of friendly bacteria, we would become nutrient deficient, and our health would suffer.

In some cases, people contain too many unfriendly bacteria and fungi, including Candida species and bacteria such as Escherichia coli or E. coli. These do not help the body gain nutrients and can, in fact, cause bloating, gut inflammation, discomfort and gas in the system. In some cases, the unfriendly bacteria lead to nonnutritive materials and food particles that are really too large to be absorbed in the system. When this happens, we develop a “leaky gut” that has been shown to cause food sensitivities and generally make us sick.

**Maintaining the Balance of Good and Bad Bacteria**

The trick to good health is to have as many of the friendly bacteria in the gut and to eliminate or reduce the numbers of unhealthy bacteria and fungi within the gut. This sets up a nice balance that prevents leaky gut syndrome and allows the digestive system to run smoothly.

But how do we do this? It turns out there are foods you can eat that contain healthy bacteria in them. Also, if you can’t eat these foods or want a simpler way to have healthy bacteria in your system, there are supplements you can take that can improve the balance of good bacteria to bad bacteria in your gut.

# Chapter 4: Whole Food Vs Refined

I don't know about you, but when it comes to our diets and nutrition, the amount of information swarming around out there is becoming overwhelming! TV commercials, books, magazine articles, social media posts and an endless stream of videos telling us which foods to eat, how much, and offering an endless parade of diet options. It's almost too much; leaving us confused about what is and isn't a good food or drink choice.

Yet, while we all seem fairly aware at this point that spinach *is* likely a healthier food choice than potato chips, a new area of focus that has emerged in recent years has more to do with the *quality* of the food rather than which food to pick.

Essentially, you've chosen to eat spinach over potato chips, but is it still good for you if it is canned, frozen, fresh, refined? This question has been a tricky one to answer which is why I wanted to shine some light on this issue and specifically how to make good choices when it comes to our food.

To begin properly, I need to define what some of these key terms mean. A *whole food* is simply a food that has not been changed in any way from its natural state. This might refer to vegetables that are grown without any modification and would be the same as if you had picked them from your own garden.

This can also refer to grains or even meat in the sense that while these foods may have been prepared by being put into a package or cut and packaged, nothing has been done that alters the food such as chemicals or preservatives added or other processes. This can be harder to ascertain, but essentially the ideal whole food would be something home-grown, picked and eaten!

By contrast, a *refined food* is a food that has had some

aspect of it removed or altered. This is not to be confused necessarily with processed foods. A *processed food* by contrast is a food that has been essentially prepared for some purpose but had nothing taken away, for example fresh orange juice that was prepared from fresh oranges, or flour from whole grain. Refined food by contrast has had a process undertaken that created a fundamental change, such as the difference that occurs when rice is converted from brown to white.

One of the key qualities when considering refined foods, is that generally speaking refined does not refer to better or improved but is often a refining process that is removing key nutrients. For example, white flour that was made from whole grain initially undergoes a process that removes a great deal of the fiber content, thus it is not as nutritionally dense or healthy as brown rice flour, as an example.

Not all refined foods are bad, as dried fruits are processed as they've had water removed but are not necessarily bad for you. Just the same, plain popcorn is refined because the heat changes its structure, but it isn't necessarily unhealthy.

One of the key takeaways then is to dig deeper into any food that may be refined or considered refined. There are many refined foods that do not deliver the nutritional benefit and have been fundamentally altered in the process such that they deliver a substantially compromised nutritional benefit. This includes products like white bread, white rice, or refined pasta as the grains used to create these products have been altered for taste and preservation and lost much of their original density.

Another example would be fruit juices that have been processed so they can be preserved and have a longer shelf life or taste sweeter. Most of these juices, whether it be apple juice, cranberry juice or otherwise have been altered and lost most of the original benefits of the actual fruits.

Thus, while you may think apple juice is just as good as eating apples, it is most certainly not! Of course, some examples would be much easier to identify, potato chips have clearly been altered from the original potatoes, just as fried chicken tenders are certainly refined from their original composition when they are still fresh.

In a perfect world of nutrition, we would only consume whole foods that go straight from farm to table. That is what I did starting in 2012, that led to my major accomplishment of ridding my body of sarcoidosis in just seven days! If you are burdened with an illness or disease, switching to whole foods would be a recommend choice for getting your body to a healthy, alkaline state. They are more nutritionally dense and will deliver the best taste and nutrition for your diet.

However, if you need to shop for refined foods, do your due diligence and determine if the refining process has fundamentally altered the food for the worse, and if so, do your best to limit them until such time you can avoid them altogether. As always, preparation equals success so do your research and eat the best food for you!

# Chapter 5:
# The Health Benefits of Probiotics

Most people spend a lot of time protecting their bodies against bacteria or getting rid of bacteria inside their lungs or gut. However, what if I told you not all bacteria is bad for you? In fact, your body relies on millions of healthy, helpful bacteria to keep you safe and healthy every day. And by giving your body beneficial probiotics, you can improve the population of helpful bacteria inside your body that are necessary for your continued health.

Eating foods rich in probiotics can not only prevent illness but also treat some disorders and imbalances. Learning which foods are high in probiotics, as well as the benefits these organisms offer to your body, will help you feel better and stay healthier over time.

## Understanding Probiotics

You have bacteria, yeast, and other microbes all over your body, both inside and out. Luckily, many of those organisms are helpful bacteria that perform vital functions for your cells, tissues, organs, and body systems.

Probiotics and the beneficial bacteria they support can help:

- Boost your immune system, allowing you to heal faster from sickness and injury.

- Prevent infection by stopping hostile bacteria from taking over.

- Improve your digestion, which allows you to better absorb nutrients from the foods you eat.

Your gut is where most of the helpful bacteria in your body lives. Keeping your digestive microflora healthy not only aids your digestion but also ensures your immune system is working properly. These two systems are directly linked.

When you throw off the balance of good versus bad bacteria in your gut, such as when you are sick or when you are taking antibiotics, you need to help your body replenish the friendly bacteria in your system. Eating probiotics can restore this balance, which creates a barrier against harmful microbes.

Probiotics and Antibiotics

Most people don't realize this but when you take antibiotics to treat an infection, you not only eliminate the bad bacteria that are making you sick but also the healthy, beneficial bacteria that can make you well. When I learned this, it no longer made sense to me to ever take antibiotics, as long as I could fix any infection issue I dealt with, with whole and natural remedies.

If you must take antibiotics, be sure to fill your body with probiotic-rich foods. When you take probiotics during and after using antibiotics, you are helping to restore the natural gut microflora that your body needs quickly. This also can help increase the effectiveness of antibiotics, which can help you feel better faster and require fewer and smaller doses of antibiotics in the future.

### *Probiotic-Rich Foods*

Foods that are cultured or fermented are good sources of probiotics, as bacteria are what create their flavor and texture. Examples of foods that are high in probiotics include cultured yogurt, miso, tempeh, kefir, buttermilk, sauerkraut, kombucha, kimchi, and nattō. While some of these foods have bacteria which grow naturally, some include bacteria added during the preparation process.

These foods and beverages contain one or more of the following strains of probiotics:

- Lactobacillus acidophilus

- Lactobacillus casei

- Bifidobacterium bifidum

- Lactobacillus bulgaricus
- Lactobacillus gasseri
- Saccharomyces boulardii
- Lactobacillus plantarum
- Bifidobacterium lactis
- Enterococcus faecium
- Bifidobacterium longum

Any food that claims to have probiotics should contain at least one of the strains listed here. This is also true for probiotic supplements, so always read the label if you are in doubt.

***Supporting a Probiotic Environment***

In addition to eating foods that contain probiotics, you

can create an environment that is supportive of the healthy bacteria in your body. You can start by altering the pH of your digestive system by eating more sour foods. Fermented vegetables and vinegars contain small amounts of probiotic, but their acid content is the most powerful part of their benefits. They contribute to a gut environment that allows probiotics to flourish.

You can also be sure the bacteria in your system have plenty of fuel by feeding them a high-fiber diet. The fermentable fiber in fresh vegetables, fruits, flax and chia seeds are perfect for giving probiotics the food they need to maintain your healthy bacteria levels.

***Eating Probiotics***

Adding probiotics to your diet is one smart move you can make to improve your health. These foods contain beneficial bacteria your body needs to fend off unwanted visitors. Help your body today by including probiotics in your next meal or snack.

# Poor Nutrition

# =

# Poor Digestion

*America stands out as the shining example of poor nutrition. There is a popular acronym used in the dietary health field and it is called SAD. This stands for Standard American Diet. Understand there is no implication that every other country has perfectly healthy diets. There are people in places all over the world suffering from the consequences of a poor diet. Often, there is little choice due to poverty.*

# Chapter 6: What Is Poor Nutrition?

In America, poor nutrition is rampant through all economic classes. Poor nutrition comes from a lack of nutrients. Poor nutrition also comes from the vast variety of processed junk foods that fill supermarket shelves and the endless options in fast food restaurants that offer quick fix meals for our fast-paced lives that overlook the main purposes of eating, nutrition!

The most obvious aspect of an unhealthy diet is an abundance of processed foods and a lack of fresh fruits, vegetables, and healthy grains. What has happened is people have created a lifestyle in which they mostly consume fast food and processed foods.

There is a common misunderstanding about what food is. The misunderstanding is that food is only something that tastes good and is eaten to fill up the stomach. This is only true if you are starving. Real food has nutritional content such as vitamins, minerals, antioxidants, fiber, healthy fats, and natural, non-processed carbohydrates.

**Poor Nutrition And Intestinal Health**

A diet low in fiber and high in saturated fats leads to constipation. Constipation is a serious issue. The body must eliminate what it digests, ideally within eight to ten hours after consumption. For this to happen, there has to be plenty of fiber in the diet and sufficient water intake. Without the right amount of fiber and water, stools become hard and it is difficult for the intestines to move them out. This causes the colon to swell as it holds feces for days or even weeks.

In order to compensate for the overload, the colon develops diverticula, which are finger-like growths stemming from the colon walls. Next diverticulitis sets in when the diverticula become infected and inflamed. According to Dr. Michael T. Murray, ND, a renowned and respected Naturopathic Physician, this leads to inflammatory bowel disease, peptic ulcers, ulcerative colitis, and other serious digestive diseases.

Nutrient absorption declines rapidly and the rest of the body suffers further disease. Doctors at Cedars-Sinai Medical Center have proven a clear link with a diet low in fibers from fruits and vegetables and colon cancer.

**Fiber Is Not All You Need**

One could take this information and assume they can simply add a fiber supplement to their diets and then they can eat all the nutritionally deficient food desired. The reality is that a balanced group of nutrients is required to maintain optimal digestive health. There are several nutrients, which are the basic essentials:

- Protein
- Healthy fats
- Carbohydrates

- Fiber
- Vitamins
- Minerals
- Water
- Antioxidants

Without all of these nutrients in proper balance, the digestive system develops toxicity and disease, further disrupting nutrient absorption. With regard to fiber, we need between 20-30 grams daily, consumed throughout the day. This fiber should come from fresh fruits, vegetables, and whole grains. The USDA recommends 5-9 full servings of whole fruits and vegetables daily.

Interestingly, when you eat 5-9 servings of vegetables and fruits daily, not only do you avoid constipation, you get plenty of vitamins, minerals, and antioxidants. The idea is to cut out processed foods and fast foods and eat whole foods in their original form.

Start to optimize your diet and get the proper nutrition. Then digestive problems can be healed. Follow a “rainbow diet.” Colorful fruits and vegetables are the ones containing high levels of antioxidants, vitamins, and minerals. The good news is that while poor nutrition contributes to digestive problems, good nutrition leads to digestive healing.

# Chapter 7: Scary Results from Eating Too Much Protein

According to statistics, most individuals in the US take in 3-5 times more protein than they need. An ideal protein intake is about 0.5 grams (500 mg) of protein per pound of lean body mass. This calculates to about 40-70 grams of protein per day. While high protein diets are extremely popular, eating excessive amounts of protein can be damaging to your health.

**The Dangers Of Eating Too Much Protein**

If you eat more protein than your body can really use, this may cause problems with your overall health and fitness in several ways.

**Too much protein can lead to these health issues:**

- Increased blood sugar
- Weight gain
- Too much body fat
- Stress on your kidneys, which must get rid of excess protein
- Loss of minerals from your bones
- Dehydration
- Cancer cell stimulation

That being said, you need to know that your body cannot live without protein. While some amino acids can be made by the body, several essential amino acids cannot be made by the body tissues, so they must be taken in through food sources. Your amino acids are what make the protein that helps grow muscle, bony tissue, enzymes, and several hormones your body needs to survive.

Your body processes protein less efficiently as you age so that eating enough high-quality protein becomes more important. You also need more protein during pregnancy so the fetus can use that protein to grow. People who are not aging or pregnant can stick to eating 40-70 grams of protein daily as suggested.

There is an upper limit as to how much protein your body can make use of. We eat, on average, much more protein than our bodies need as well as too much carbohydrate-containing foods and not enough foods high in healthy fat.

Part of the problem is that the consumption of meat has risen to a great degree in the last century. Most of this meat is not high-quality meat and comes from animal farms where animals are fed grains that have been genetically altered instead of grass in a pasture. Until you can wean yourself away from meat, be sure to eat meat that has been pasture-fed. But even this can still lead to protein excesses in the body.

**What Protein Does In Your Body**

When you eat protein, your body takes what it needs and converts all of the rest of it into sugar and finally into fat. When your blood sugar levels are increased from eating too much protein, you put yourself at risk of getting infections by yeast (called Candidiasis) and pathogenic bacteria. The growth of cancer cells is stimulated by the excesses of sugar and fat in your body.

There is a biochemical pathway known as the mammalian target of rapamycin that is stimulated by having too much protein in your system. This pathway plays a role in cancer formation. In order to avoid stimulating the pathway, you need to keep your protein levels to the proper amounts.

Eating too much protein causes stress on the kidneys. The kidneys are responsible for removing the nitrogenous waste products in the bloodstream and when there is too much protein, both the excess protein and water is lost through the kidneys, resulting in dehydration. This was proven in a research study that involved athletes who engaged in endurance sports.

## The Proper Amount of Protein May Prolong Your Life

There have been recent research studies that relate to calorie restriction and longevity. In particular, restriction of protein intake leads to a longer life, particularly restriction of the amino acid known as methionine. This is found in high levels in meats. Other research indicates that the balance of amino acids might be the most important factor in gaining a long life.

## Calculating The Amount Of Protein You Need

You need to know exactly how much protein you need to consume in order to be healthy. It can be calculated as taking in 500 mg of protein per pound of lean body mass or about 40-60 grams of protein daily. If you are excessively exercising or are pregnant, you need to take in about 25 percent more than that.

You also need to remember that a serving of protein is about the size of one deck of cards. Then you need to estimate the amount of protein you need. Your lean body mass is your percent body fat subtracted from one hundred. Make that into a percentage and multiply that by your total weight in pounds. Multiply that number into 0.5 grams per pound to get your protein requirement for the day.

### What Foods To Eat

To get the protein you need, but not too much, choose protein found in free-range eggs, meat from farm-fed animals only, fish from pristine waters, legumes, seeds, and nuts. Forty grams of protein isn't really very much: about two hamburger patties. Read food labels and look up the amount of protein in the foods you are eating. If you are eating too much, just adjust your diet so you are eating the right amount of protein.

# Spices & Foods That Are Great For The Gut

*You may or may not realize it but there is no shortage of spices and food that are healthy for, and helpful to, the digestive system. There is, however, a shortage of knowledge about those things. The number of whole, plant-based foods I could share here would have me writing 'til the cows come home (and of course, never to MY home). So, to save me all that writing, I am just going to share two. One food item from the vegetable family and one food item from the fruit family. But first, herbs must take center stage.*

# Chapter 8:
# 10 Herbs That Improve Digestion

When most people think of the term digestion, they assume it has to do with what goes on in the stomach- and that's the end.

While this belief isn't wrong per se, as we are taught this in high school, a more complete picture of digestion entails what happens to the food from the time we eat it, to when it's excreted.

As such, efficient digestion promotes the maximum uptake of nutrients, so what we have left is basically just plain ole' poop

**So What Can You Do If You Suspect Something Is Amiss With Your Digestion?**

Luckily, nature gifted us many effective remedies

to successfully combat digestive issues- whether it be relating to poor absorption, reflux disease or constipation- there is something for everyone.

**Turmeric**

Long been used in Asia, more specifically Indian regions, Turmeric has been shown to decrease the incidence of peptic ulcer disease. Turmeric contains the compound curcumin, which is a potent antioxidant and anti-inflammatory. This effect significantly reduces the chance of ulceration occurring in the stomach, typically from an inflamed region exposed to strong gastric acid.

**Cinnamon**

Used frequently as a spice for flavor, cinnamon is also effective in treating gas and associated bloating. Cinnamon has also traditionally been used as treatment for upset stomach, and to stimulate appetite.

**Aloe Vera**

The uses of aloe Vera for digestive health is unmatched

by any other herb. Aloe Vera contains tons of amino acids, vitamins and enzymes, which help to speed up digestion and fecal transit. Aloe Vera also boosts immunity and, is a natural anti-fungal and antibiotic, and is useful in management of inflamed intestines and the colon. Taking aloe in gel form is the most popular method of use.

**Cardamom**

An essential component of the spice Garam Masala, it is frequently used in Indian dishes, especially curry. Cardamom can be used to stimulate appetite, reduce bloating, and treat heartburn and constipation, making it a very versatile herb.

**Chia Seeds**

As if there was nothing more this superfood could accomplish, chia seeds help promote normal intestinal transit of food as well as exerting anti-inflammatory effects in the intestinal tract.

### Slippery Elm Bark

A Native American remedy used for centuries, it becomes a very thick, viscous gel when combined with water. It is especially efficient at soothing irritated segments of the digestive tract, making it very useful intreating irritable bowel syndrome.

### Peppermint

A popular ingredient in many herbal remedies to treat gas and indigestion. In fact, a study conducted in 2011 demonstrated that peppermint is effective in managing pain associated with irritable bowel syndrome, since it has the ability to regulate pain pathways in the intestine. It however, will not help to reduce gastric reflux.

### Ginger

Ginger promotes complete digestion and subsequent absorption of foods, as well as being useful in the treatment of nausea and indigestion. Ginger also helps relieve the pain from intestinal colic, by slowing down the frequency or intensity of spasms.

**Dandelion**

Dandelion, one of the most widely used bitter herbs can decrease the likelihood of experiencing indigestion since it speeds up gastric motility, or the movement of food from the stomach into the intestines. Dandelion also helps in the absorption of fat, since it stimulates the production of bile.

**Burdock Root**

This is a useful herbal preparation especially for people that struggle with sluggish digestion, or reduced stomach acid production. Burdock root helps with digestion by stimulating the production of more gastric acid- but caution needs to be followed, as it is not for everyone. If you have a history of gastric reflux or irritable bowel syndrome, Burdock Root can exacerbate them.

# Chapter 9: Anatomy of Brussels Sprouts

You may remember Brussels sprouts as those small, round veggies that ended up on your plate as a child, or in the pet dog's mouth. Like most children, you probably didn't want to eat them or cringed at the way they smelled while cooking. Despite these little drawbacks, however, they were put on your plate for good reason: they're actually one of the world's healthiest foods, making them a diet necessity.

Those little veggies that look like mini cabbages more than anything are packed with vitamins and minerals that can do wonders for your body and your immune system. Not only are they highly nutritious, but they're also extremely versatile and can be prepared in a number of different ways. This means you have a variety of options for how to add them to your diet, so you won't ever get bored with these perfectly crafted vegetables made by nature with the utmost care.

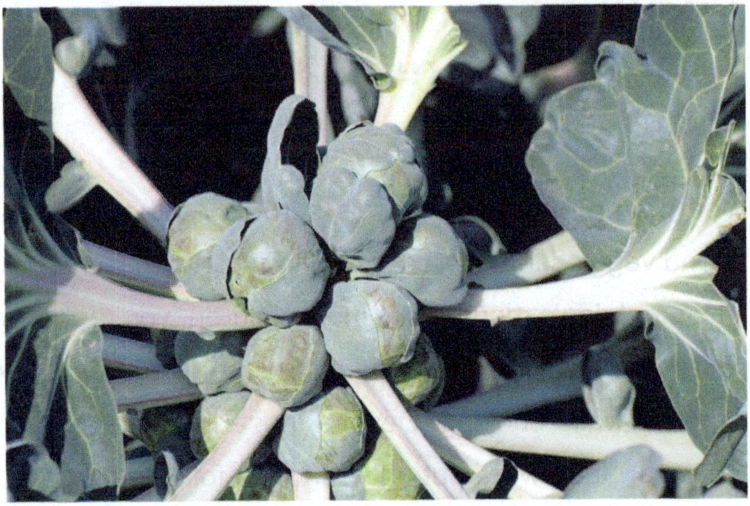

**What Are Brussels Sprouts?**

Brussels sprouts don't just look like mini cabbages; they're actually members of the Gemmifera Group of cabbages. These cabbages are grown for their edible buds and may have gotten their name from Brussels, Belgium, where they are believed to have originated and are highly popular. Ancestors of the modern Brussels sprout were most likely cultivated in ancient Rome, but the sprouts we know and love today were likely grown as early as the 13th century in Belgium. A small, leafy vegetable, Brussels sprouts are packed with protein, vitamins, fiber and many more nutrients.

A staple of Belgium for many years, Brussels sprouts have found popularity due to their high nutritional value and versatility in the kitchen.

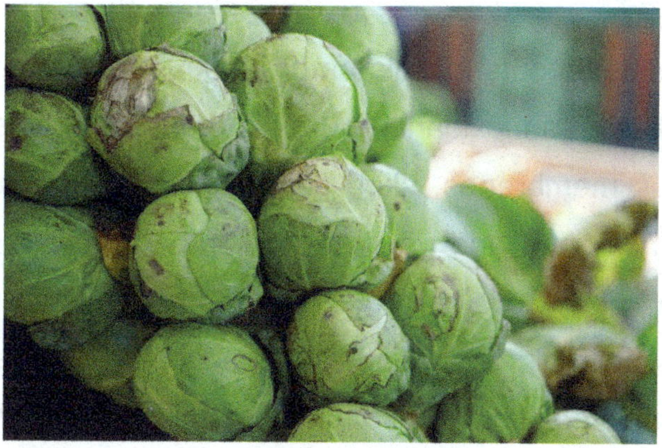

**Nutritional Value And Health Benefits**

No matter how they come, Brussels sprouts can offer you an excellent source of nutrients. Packed with good things from the earth and nature, these vegetables are perfectly crafted to maintain health and wellness. When raw, Brussels sprouts are an excellent source of vitamin

C and K and contain good amounts of B vitamins such as vitamin B6, folic acids, and other essential minerals. They are also a good source of protein and dietary fiber and contain absolutely no cholesterol. Like cabbages, they may cause an overactive bowel if eaten too much, so it is important to eat them in moderation. More than making you extra-regular, they can also cause gas and bloating if eaten too much.

Brussels sprouts are also a great source of vitamin A, which is an antioxidant required for maintaining healthy mucus membranes, skin, and promoting optimal eye health. Foods and veggies rich with vitamin A have been known to offer protection against some cancers such as oral cavity and lung cancer. The extent of cancer-protection in Brussels sprouts is still widely researched, but promising findings hint that this veggie helps fight cancer causing agents and cleanses the body of many toxins.

Brussels sprouts are also one of the leading veggie sources of vitamin K, which is best for bone health and preventing diseases and disorders of the bones such as osteoporosis. In addition to these nutrients, Brussels sprouts are an excellent source of the following minerals: copper, iron, manganese, calcium, potassium, and phosphorus.

Unlike some grains and other plant-based foods, Brussels sprouts are not necessarily used for specific problems. This is because they are so rich in vitamin and minerals—they are simply a highly nutritious addition to any diet.

As already mentioned, Brussels sprouts help with a number of health problems and provide the body with the support it needs to build strong bones, remove toxins and cancer-causing radicals and agents, regulate metabolism, promote strong muscles, oxygenate the blood, and do much, much more. These superfoods are a do-it-all veggie that promotes optimal health and wellbeing.

**How They're Prepared**

Adding Brussels sprouts to your diet is incredibly

easy because they can be prepared so many different ways. Oven roasted Brussels sprouts; stir-fried, baked, shredded sprouts, parmesan sprouts, breaded, and raw sprouts are just a few ways to prepare these veggies. There are many oven roasted recipes that can be made with onions and fresh garlic.

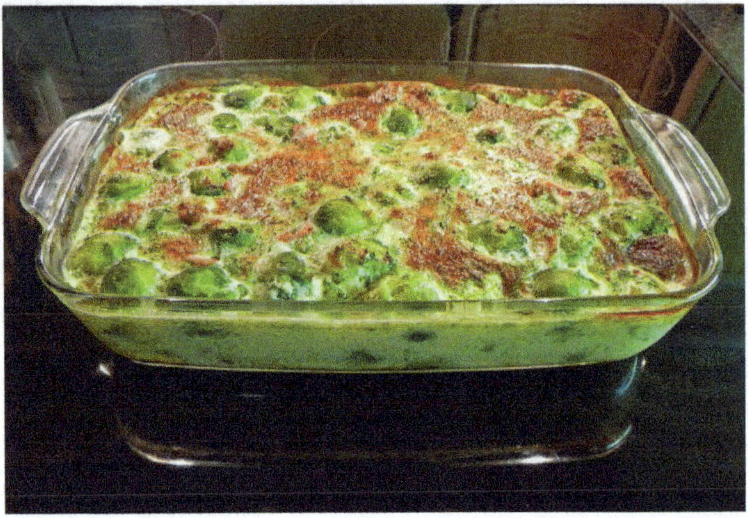

They can also be added to soups, salads, casseroles, pasta dishes, vegetable loafs, and used as garnish around poultry and fish. There's truly no right or wrong way to make these, so simply find a recipe that intrigues you and get cooking!

**Created By Nature, Made for You**

Though Brussels sprouts may have gotten a bad reputation when you were a child, you can now look at them with new eyes. These little vegetables are wholly good for you with only benefits for your body and wellbeing. When eaten in moderation, these beauties will keep you regular, have you feeling great, and inspire you to create a healthy diet around them and their health benefits. Mom always said, eat your vegetables, and she was right!

# Chapter 10: Cherry, Cherry Bo Berry. . .

Have you ever heard of the cherry diet? It's becoming as popular these days as that cutesy little name-rhyming song we learned as children. What makes this diet so popular is that it's incredibly easy to follow. There is only one rule to this diet – to eat cherries every day and/or to drink fresh cherry juice. That's it!

Although they are more popular for their taste, researchers are now seeing that cherries are actually extremely healthy as well. The bioactive components and nutrients found in this fruit are linked to the prevention of diabetes, cardiovascular disease, inflammatory diseases, cancer, and Alzheimer's disease.

However, not only will they protect you from various health conditions, but cherries will also make it easier for you to accomplish your weight-loss goals.

**There are a few reasons why cherries help promote weight loss.**

First of all, they don't contain a lot of calories (the average cherry contains 5 calories). Although a lot of other fruits contain fewer calories, it's worth noting that cherries aren't considered to be high-calorie foods. You can easily satisfy your hunger with a dozen cherries, which roughly amounts to 60 calories.

Cherries do a good job of satisfying your hunger because they are rich in fiber. All weight-loss diets that exist suggest that you should consume more fiber, since this nutrient isn't easily digested by your body. In other words, you will have to drink a lot of water in order to move it through your digestive system. This will help you with your weight loss goals because water will contribute to the feeling of fullness.

It's also worth mentioning that many people often confuse thirst with hunger, so staying hydrated will also prevent you from overeating. The great thing about fiber is that consuming it will help you feel full for an extended time period. This means it will actually help prevent you from overeating on other foods that are potentially high in calories.

On top of that, the soluble type of fiber that absorbs water helps you by slowing the absorption of sugars, thus making your body store less fat.

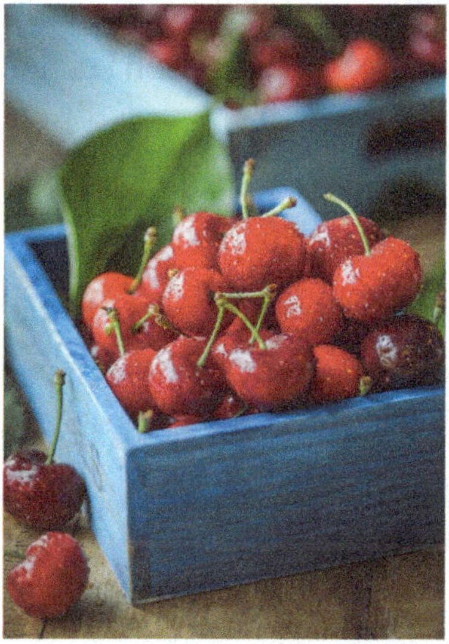

Dark cherries also contain compounds known as anthocyanins, which will help you reduce belly fat. Back in 2008, the Journal of Agricultural and Food Chemistry published a study, which showed just how powerful these compounds are when it comes to reduced belly fat.

Anthocyanins are flavonoid pigments found in a lot of different fruits and vegetables. Although there is still a lot of research to be done on the way anthocyanins are absorbed and distributed in the tissues of our bodies, researchers generally agree that these compounds can be a powerful tool for weight loss.

**Can Dark Cherries Reduce Belly Fat?**

Although cherries can definitely help you reduce belly fat, simply adding them to your existing diet won't do the trick. There are no magical foods that you will help you shed those extra pounds simply by consuming them.

Cherries will help you reach your weight loss goals, but you will also need to make sure that your diet is filled with other fresh produce. On top of that, you should avoid eating junk food and you should exercise regularly if you want to shed those extra pounds.

With that being said, you should definitely include cherries into your dietary regimen, and you should be encouraged to consume them whenever you feel the urge to snack on something. By keeping your fridge stocked with washed cherries, you will always have a healthy snack that you can munch on.

# 40 Tips for Eating Healthy

# While Eating Out

*Let's face it, like most you probably lead a very busy life. You likely don't always have time after you get home from a long day at work to cook or you may just be too tired to do so. With a restaurant on almost every corner, it can be very tempting to go out for a meal or get takeout to bring home. That's ok because restaurants have some great food and dining out is also a great way to unwind and de-stress after a hard day at work.*

***But what if you want to maintain a healthy diet?***

*The trick is to find ways to eat out in a healthy way and this is definitely possible. Here are some helpful tips on ways to eat healthy when dining out. These helpful tips will allow you to enjoy going out to restaurants without sacrificing your healthy lifestyle. The bottom line is to make smart and mindful choices and enjoy!*

# Chapter 11:
# Eating Out – Information Is Key

### 1. Don't Be Shy

Many people are guilty about not wanting to "rock the boat" when they are out eating and ask too many questions because they don't want to be seen as a high maintenance customer. You need to put yourself first and ask all the questions you need to in order to obtain a truly healthy meal for yourself.

### 2. Ask How A Certain Menu Item Is Prepared

It's pretty obvious how fried chicken is prepared but with other entrees that may not be the case. So, ask your waiter how certain dishes are prepared and if there are any healthy alternative cooking methods. If you are trying to eat healthy, it won't help if that innocent sounding dish you ordered is actually sautéed in loads of butter.

### 3. Look For Heart Healthy Items

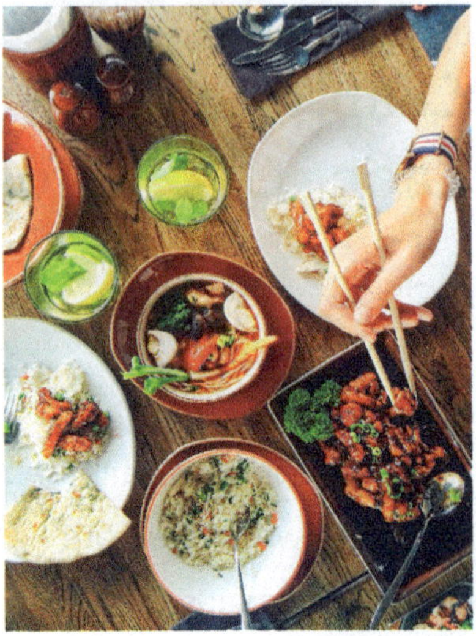

Even fast food chains are starting to recognize the trend of many consumers toward healthier eating. Many times menu items that are healthier and lower calorie choices will be indicated by a heart stamp next to their name. So, choose these over that beer battered fish with tartar sauce.

### 4. Ask For Calorie Counts And Ingredient Information On A Dish

As people get more health conscious when they eat at restaurants, these same restaurants are starting to realize that they must be proactive in giving more information about the food they prepare if they want to attract a wide variety of customers. Many restaurants are now disclosing calorie information, as they are required to by laws and regulations, so take advantage of this when ordering.

### 5. Protein And Produce Should Be The Focus Of Your Menu Search

If you look at a menu with your mind wide open, you are most likely going to pick your meal based on impulse or cravings and this can easily lead to making unhealthy choices. If you change the way you approach looking at the menu and already have in mind that you want a protein-based entrée with vegetables, you will focus on this and are more likely to pick a healthy entrée from the menu.

### 6. Ask If They Have Half Portions

Restaurants do not advertise it but many actually have what they call a ½ portion. They may cost more, but are a good way to not eat too much of an unhealthy meal and will still save you some money too. Another great option to maintain portion control is to order from the appetizer menu instead of the entrée menu, as the portions will be much smaller.

### 7. Don't Be Duped

You always like to think that the eating places you patronize are totally above board or in the know when it comes to their food but that simply is not always the case. Sometimes a restaurant's so called "healthy entrees" may not really be all that healthy. Therefore, try not to be fooled; do your research.

### 8. Hold It Right There

One of the best ways to eat healthy when dining out is to tell your waiter or waitress exactly how you want your meal prepared. It's ok to say hold the butter, no sauce on top please, and hold the cheese. Additionally, you can ask for meats to be unseasoned or unsalted if you are watching your sodium intake.

### 9. Indulge Smartly

Everyone deserves to spoil themselves once in a while

so, you shouldn't shame yourself if you indulge every so often and order what you consider a real treat even though it's a little unhealthy. Moderation is key. The trick is indulging smartly by doing things such as eating less of the entrée and making sure, you order healthy sides with it to compensate for the unhealthy portion of the meal.

**10. Look At The Menu Online**

One great way to eat healthy is to decide what you will order before you go to a restaurant to eat. That way you will be less influenced by such things as aroma and looking what other patrons have ordered when you are at the restaurant

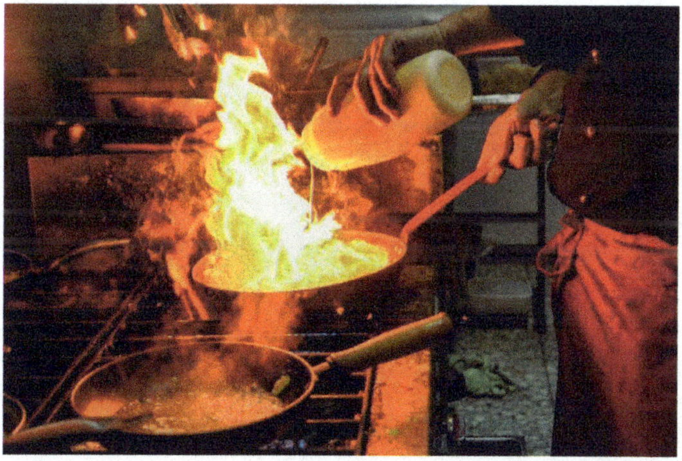

### 11. Avoid Establishments With Limited Menus

Sure, pizza houses and custom burger joints have some great eats but they are also places that have very few if any healthy menu choices. Beware of these types of places when you want to go out for dinner but still eat healthy. Also beware of food prepared at super high temperatures. When the chemicals in foods mix with high temperatures, it causes carcinogens to form (cancer causing agents).

# Chapter 12:
# Eating Out – Innovative Ideas

### 1. Watch For Hidden Fats

Traditional foods such as Thai foods are generally good for you but can hide fat in some of their dishes. Watch for foods that are prepared in such things as low-grade fatty oils. They may not look like it but they can be very unhealthy. Sushi is another healthy food that often has unhealthy mayo hidden in its dips.

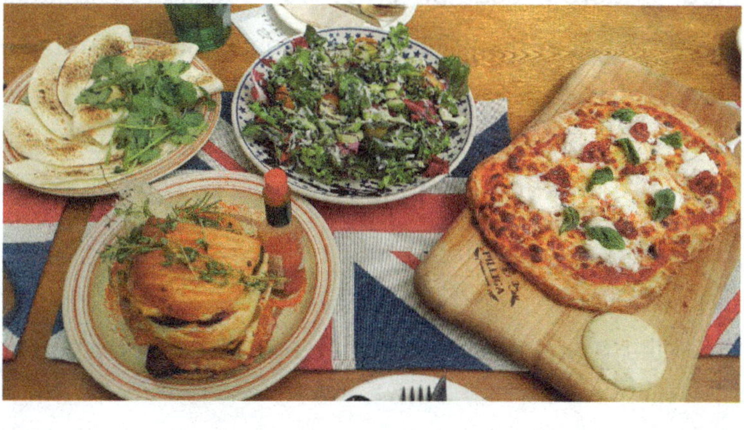

## 13. Substitutes Are OK

Many restaurants will let you mix or substitute the sides that come with your entree. Try selecting a fruit as opposed to macaroni and cheese or French fries. Get foods such as chicken in a skinless baked version instead of fried with the skin on. Even little things like using a nut milk instead of cream in your coffee will pay big health benefits over time.

## 14. Look For Clues That A Food Is Unhealthy

They are a few words associated with food dishes that should send up a big red flag that they are unhealthy. Avoid foods that have the words au gratin, braised, fried, buttered, scampi, creamed, escalloped in their titles, and also avoid cheese, cream, and Hollandaise sauces.

## 15. Watch For These Clues To Foods Being Healthier Too

Just like there are words that are red flags when it

comes to unhealthy eating there are also words that will give you the green light to go ahead and eat them too. If a food has the words baked, roasted, broiled, poached, or steamed in its title then it will likely be a fairly healthy choice. *Garden Fresh* is another good indicator phrase too.

**16. Avoid Too Much Sodium**

A little bit of salt is good for you but too much is a definite no-no. Be careful of such things as pickled foods, and foods that are smoked. In addition, soy sauce, soup broths, and teriyaki sauce can really significantly increase your salt intake.

# Chapter 13: Eating Out – Just Good Advice

### 17. Seek Out Whole Grains

Whole grains tend to be a much healthier choice when it comes to such things as sandwiches, breads, and pizza crust. Have a whole-wheat tortilla instead of a regular one the next time you are eating out and order brown rice instead of plain white rice if possible.

### 18. Eat Fish

Fish (except the fried variety) is always a great choice as it is naturally low in fat and has beneficial omega-3 fatty acids too.

### 19. Lean Meat Rule – Avoid Saturated Fats

Sure, that ½-pound house specialty burger probably

tastes amazing but your heart will skip a beat or two when it is placed in front of you because it's so unhealthy. Tenderloin of beef or pork, seafood and poultry make excellent lean choices as long as they are not covered in fatty sauces.

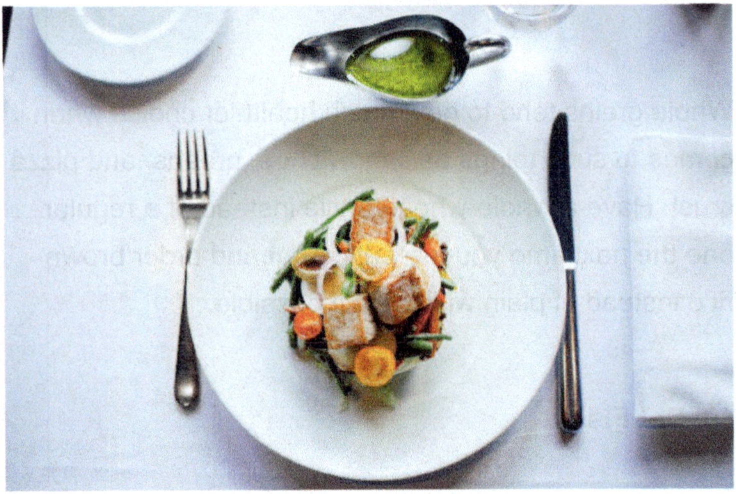

**20. Be Mindful Of What You Are Eating**

Don't just eat; enjoy the food you eat too. If you are more conscious of such things as aroma, flavor, and texture, it's a proven fact that you will be much more likely to stop when you are satisfied versus over stuffed, which always means you ate too much.

### 21. Tomato Sauce Over Cream Sauce

This one is for Italian food lovers. When it comes to eating healthy, 99% of the time a tomato sauce is a much healthier option for you than a cream-based pasta sauce because tomato sauce varieties are much lower in calories, like in the hundreds.

### 22. Don't Sit Next To The Kitchen

If you are trying to decide what to order and a parade of unhealthy entrees is passing by you every minute you might have trouble sticking to your guns in ordering a healthy meal. So, if the restaurant tries to put you near the kitchen, ask to be moved somewhere else. This is especially true if they want to seat you near the desert case.

# Chapter 14: Eating Out – The More The Merrier

### 23. Share Deserts

Deserts are an awesome way to end any delicious meal; unfortunately, they are loaded with sugar, calories, fat, calories, and other eating undesirables. Go ahead and indulge but share it with others instead of eating it all yourself. Limit your intake to 2 or 3 bites every time.

### 24. Split Meals

Most restaurants serve extremely large portions, which leads to overeating and taking in way more calories than you need. Avoid this by sharing a meal with your significant other or a friend. Not only will it make for healthier eating but it will save you some money too.

### 25. Even A Pizza Can Be Healthy

They is no reason to avoid pizza when eating out because you can order it in a healthy way. Do such things as ordering thin crust, loading on the veggies, and avoiding the high calorie, high fat meat toppings. Another good idea is asking for more sauce and less cheese and by all means limit your portion to a maximum of two slices.

### 26. Don't Order Individual Appetizers

Everyone likes to spoil themselves with an appetizer once in a while when eating out. The problem is most appetizers are not the healthiest of choices. Additionally, most people will order an appetizer and the main dish, which leads to a high caloric overload. So instead of gobbling down an appetizer or two yourself, share them among your group, have a couple of bites and then stop.

# Chapter 15: Eating Out – Don't Overlook The Obvious

## 27. Avoid Fried Foods At All Costs

Everyone knows how bad fried foods are for you. Sure they taste great, many foods that are bad for you do; but do yourself a favor and resist the urge to say it's ok to get fried food tonight. Pick a much healthier prepared dish instead because you will still enjoy it and gain the health benefits too.

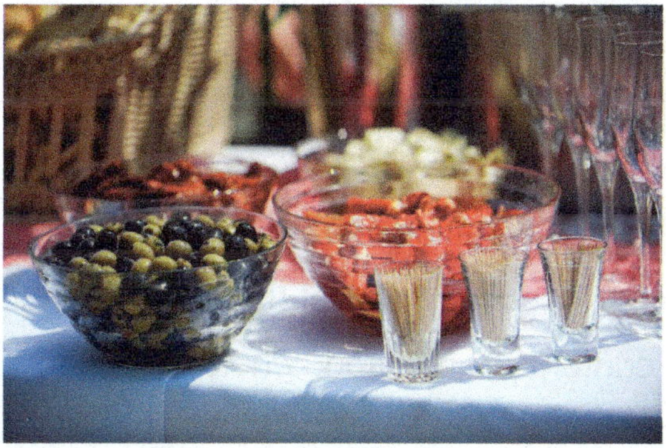

## 28. Don't Overeat

Many times, you or someone you go out to eat with will order appetizers, an entrée, and dessert. When you do things like this you feel compelled to eat every little bit because you paid for it. So don't order so much food. You will be healthier because of it and also not be uncomfortably stuffed the rest of the night. Keep in mind you can take as much as you want to go, andmake several meals out of the leftovers.

## 29. Go Gourmet

If you can afford it, gourmet food is usually a healthy choice. They are known for smaller and more natural type portions where the emphasis is on the flavor and not on the amount of food, you eat.

## 30. Avoid Buffets

Buffets are an invitation to eat as unhealthy as possible. It is mass produced food that usually is very high in salt and fat content. In addition, when is the last time you walked into a buffet and a member of your party didn't say, "I am going to get my money's worth tonight." The temptation to over eat in these places is huge so it's better just to avoid them altogether.

### 31. Order First

How many times have you been to a restaurant and changed your order after you placed it? The answer is probably not very many. So in order to eat healthy without being influenced by others during the ordering process, volunteer to place your order first.

# Chapter 16:
# Eating Out – Healthy Ideas

### 32. Get Sauces On The Side

Sauces are generally not the healthiest choice in eating for sure but they do make a dish taste good. When your food comes with the sauce already poured over it, you lose control over the portion and you pretty much don't have a choice but to eat all of it. You can cut down on the amount of that unhealthy sauce you eat by asking your waiter to put it on the side instead.

### 33. Use A Fork For Salad Dressings

There are not many foods that are healthier for you when eating out than that side salad you get with your meal; that is until it is smothered in fatty dressing. Get the dressing on the side and dip your fork in it for just the right amount of flavor and portion control instead of getting it poured over top by the restaurant where the vegetables will be drowning in it.

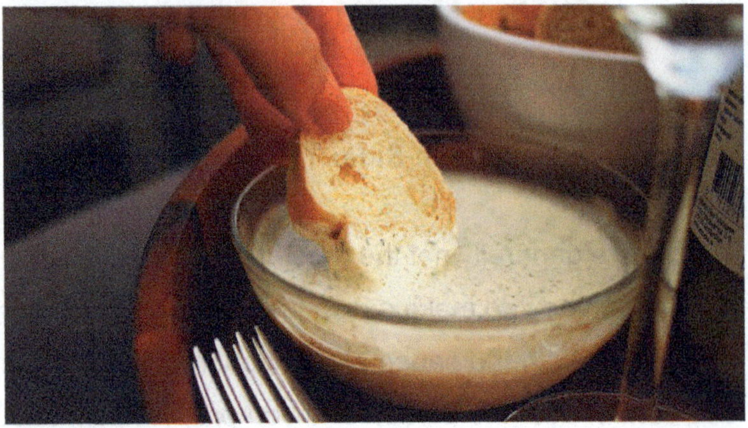

**34. Drink Water**

Everyone enjoys a beer, soda or glass of sweet tea with their meal but you are loading up on calories and unhealthy sugar when doing it. Get a healthy glass of water instead and your body will thank you. At the very least, limit yourself to just one beverage with your meal.

### 35. Ask For More Vegetables

Unless they are drowned in butter or have fatty meats added into them, vegetables are usually both a healthy and low-calorie alternative when eating out. So don't be afraid to ask for a double helping of vegetables instead of that fully loaded baked potato.

### 36. Send Back The Free Munchies

When was the last time you *didn't* have a piece of bread or a few chips at restaurant after they were set down in front of you while you were waiting for your meal? Throw in some butter or some dip and it can lead to some pretty unhealthy calorie loaded pre-meal eats. Resist the temptation and politely decline them as they are placed in front of you.

# Chapter 17:
# Eating Out – Get Creative

## 37. Get A Before Meal Doggy Bag

It has been mentioned before that many restaurants will serve portions that are double or triple the size that you would normally eat at home. If that is typical of a favorite restaurant you frequent, have them box half of the serving BEFORE you start digging into it.

## 38. Eat Less Of The "Real Thing"

If you have a craving for something like some good old fashioned ice cream, don't substitute and get frozen yogurt instead. Research shows this will not leave your craving satisfied and you will just look to eat more. Instead, settle for a lesser amount of the real thing instead.

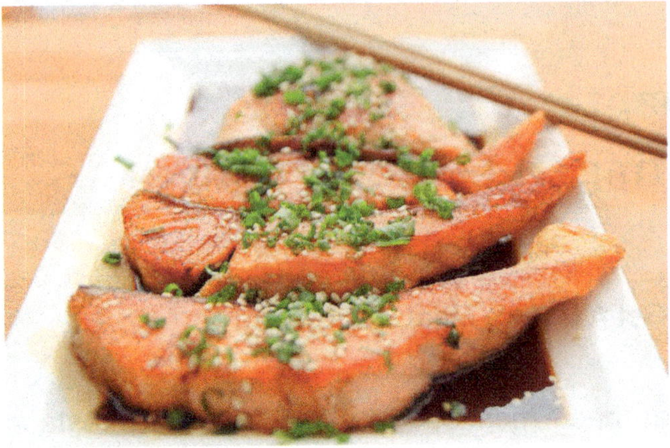

### 39. Eat A Healthy Snack Before Going Out To Dinner

This may sound a little crazy but its purpose is twofold. One, you will not feel famished so you will better resist the temptation to over-order the amount of food you get. Two, you will have healthy eating already on your mind while ordering.

### 40. Make A Reservation If Possible

Having to wait for a table at a restaurant can lead to feeling famished and that leads to mindless eating and overeating. Additionally, there is the danger of having a few drinks and some greasy appetizers while waiting for your table to become available. To help avoid this, make reservations.

# Natural Remedies

# To Get Relief

# Chapter 18 :
# Relief From Celiac Disease

Celiac is an autoimmune disorder that affects the digestive system. People with celiac disease cannot eat gluten, a protein found in wheat, rye and barley, because it will damage their small intestine. When gluten is ingested, the immune system reacts by attacking the lining of the small intestine, which can lead to nutrient malabsorption and other problems.

Symptoms of celiac disease can vary from person to person, and may include gastrointestinal issues like abdominal pain, bloating, diarrhea and constipation, as well as fatigue, headache, anemia and skin rashes.

While there is currently no cure for celiac disease, there are a few natural remedies that may help to lessen the symptoms. These include eliminating gluten from the diet, taking probiotics supplements, consuming omega-3 fatty acids, and taking a multivitamin. Some people also find relief by taking digestive enzymes or herbal supplements like L-glutamine or slippery elm bark.

What does following a gluten-free diet look like? This means avoiding all foods that contain gluten, which is a protein found in wheat, barley, and rye. Probiotics are beneficial bacteria that can help improve gut health. Taking a multivitamin can help ensure that you are getting all the nutrients you need while following a gluten-free diet.

Consulting with a naturopathic doctor or a licensed nutritionist can help you to develop a personalized treatment plan that will work best for you.

# Chapter 19: Relief From Crohn's Disease

Crohn's disease is a type of inflammatory bowel disease (IBD) that can affect any part of the gastrointestinal tract from mouth to anus. Symptoms may include abdominal pain, diarrhea, vomiting, weight loss, fever, and other symptoms. Bowel obstruction and perforation are potential complications.

Crohn's is thought to be caused by an abnormal response by the body's immune system to normal gut bacteria. If left untreated by natural methods, medications or in some more severe cases surgery, Crohn's could increase your risk for other health problems.

There is no one-size-fits-all fix for Crohn's disease as symptoms may vary widely from person to person. However, some natural remedies that have been shown to be helpful for Crohn's disease include:

1) Probiotics: Probiotics are beneficial bacteria that can help improve gut health and reduce inflammation. Some good probiotic strains to try include Lactobacillus and Bifidobacterium.

2) Omega-3 fatty acids: Omega-3 fatty acids are anti-inflammatory and can help reduce inflammation in the gut. Sources of omega-3 fatty acids include fish oil supplements, flaxseed oil, and chia seeds.

3) Herbs: Turmeric and ginger and curcumin. Curcumin is the active yellow pigment in turmeric. It possesses remarkable beneficial anti-oxidant, anti-inflammatory, anti-cancer, and neuroprotective properties.

# Chapter 20: Relief From Gallbladder Disease

The gallbladder is a small organ located just below the liver that stores bile, a digestive fluid that helps to break down fat. Bile is released from the gallbladder into the digestive tract through a small tube called the common bile duct.

Gallbladder disease is a condition that results if the gallbladder doesn't function properly. When that happens, bile can back up and cause inflammation and damage to the gallbladder and other organs in the area. Gallbladder disease can lead to various symptoms, including pain in the upper right abdomen, nausea, vomiting, and jaundice. Treatment for gallbladder disease depends on its underlying cause. Surgery may

There are different types of gallbladder disease, and therefore there is no one-size-fits-all natural remedy. However, some general lifestyle and diet changes may help to ease symptoms and improve overall gallbladder function.

Cutting back on fatty foods, consuming more fiber-rich foods and staying hydrated by drinking plenty of water are all important dietary changes to make. Adding in Garcinia cambogia extract, artichoke leaf extract or milk thistle may also help to improve gallbladder health.

Regular exercise is also beneficial for overall health and can help reduce the risk of developing gallstones. Finally, managing stress levels is important as chronic stress can lead to increased inflammation throughout the body, causing additional health risks.

# Chapter 21: Relief From Ulcerative Colitis Disease

As mentioned earlier, the colon is one of your hollow organs and is part of the large intestine. It is a long, coiled tube that removes water and wastes from the body.

Ulcerative colitis (UC) is a debilitating and often painful condition that affects the colon. It is typically diagnosed using a combination of medical history, physical examination, blood tests, stool tests, X-rays or endoscopy. In people with UC, the lining of the colon becomes inflamed causing ulcers to form on the surface. This can lead to fatigue, rectal bleeding, diarrhea, abdominal pain and cramps, and weight loss.

There is no cure for UC, and symptoms can vary, but there are treatments available to help manage the symptoms and prevent flare-ups. If you have UC, it's important to work with your nutritionist, Registered Dietitian (RD), or doctor to create a treatment plan that works for you. These treatments may include anti-inflammatory medications, immunosuppressive drugs, diet changes, or surgery.

Some herbs and spices that may be helpful for ulcerative colitis include ginger, licorice, boswellia, curcumin, and chamomile. Each of these herbs has anti-inflammatory properties that can help to reduce UC symptoms.

Additionally, keeping a food diary can be helpful in identifying triggers causing the flare-ups. Nightshade vegetables such as tomatoes, potatoes, and peppers are common triggers for many people with UC. Avoiding or reducing intake of these vegetables can help to control symptoms. Working with a professional who specializes in gastrointestinal disorders can be extremely helpful in developing an individualized diet plan that works for you.

# Conclusion

***The Road To A Healthy Gut***

*When the friendly bacteria vastly outnumber the unfriendly bacteria, your gut will run smoothly, you will get the nutrients you need from the metabolism of the good bacteria, and you will generally aid in good health and proper nutrition.*

*Start to optimize your diet and get the proper nutrition. Then digestive problems can be healed. Follow a "rainbow diet." Colorful fruits and vegetables are the ones containing high levels of antioxidants, vitamins, and minerals. Good nutrition leads to digestive healing.*

# Appendix A

## Grocery List Of Foods That Are Great For The Gut

1. Almonds
2. Apples
3. Apricots
4. Artichokes
5. Asparagus
6. Avocados
7. Bananas
8. Beans and Lentils
9. Beets
10. Bell Peppers
11. Berries
12. Broccoli
13. Brussels Sprouts
14. Cabbage
15. Cantaloupe
16. Carrots
17. Cauliflower
18. Cherries

19. Chia

20. Coconut

21. Dark Chocolate

22. Eggs

23. Fish

24. Flax Seeds

25. Garlic

26. Grapes

27. Hot Peppers

28. Kale Greens

29. Kiwi

30. Lemons and Limes

31. Low-Fat Yogurt and Kefir

32. Mangoes

33. Mushrooms

34. Oats

35. Olive Oil

36. Oranges

37. Papaya

38. Peaches

39. Pineapple

40. Pumpkin

41. Pomegranates

42. Quinoa

43. Spinach

44. Spirulina

45. Sprouts

46. Sweet Potatoes

47. Swiss Chard Greens

48. Tomatoes

49. Walnuts

50. Wild Caught Salmon

Of course, there are more great and nutritious foods to add to your cart, but this is a great place to start. Happy shopping!

# Appendix B
# How can Terri help me?

Congratulations on completing this book! What God has for YOU is for YOU. You are fully capable of doing great things according to God's plans and purposes for your life, and your willingness to act.

If I may ask you a few questions, your responses could prove to be a helpful on-going guidepost for your journey. Simply fill in the scorecard below being brutally honest with yourself. This is for *your* improvement, so answer as though you are serious about improving.

Once completed, if you would like coaching with a tiny bit of handholding as you begin your transformation, take a screenshot of your completed scorecard and email it to me at terri@lawofraw.com. Be sure to include your name and best contact phone number. For the Subject, put: "I want to fix my gut"

Someone from my office will get back to you as soon as possible to set up a time to meet. After all, everyone could use a little help now and then.

What is my vision/mission for my health?

______________________________________________

______________________________________________

______________________________________________

______________________________________________

_________________________________________

1. What actions can I put in place to help me stay on track with my vision/mission?

______________________________________________

______________________________________________

______________________________________________

______________________________________________

_________________________

2. What take-ways from this book will help move me to act?

________________________________________

________________________________________

________________________________________

________________________________________

3. Yes, I desire a one-on-one consultation to help me conquer the following health goals.

a. ______________________________

b. ______________________________

c. ______________________________

d. ______________________________

# Appendix C
# Changes I Will Make to Improve My Health

________________________________________

________________________________________

________________________________________

________________________________________

________________________________________

________________________________________

________________________________________

**My Plans of Action to Achieve Those Changes**

Step 1

Step 2

Step 3

____________________________________________

____________________________________________

____________________________________________

____________________________________________

I am assigning ________________________________ as my accountability partner to ensure I do all three steps listed to achieve my health goal(s). Be sure to select someone who really will keep you on your toes!

# About The Author

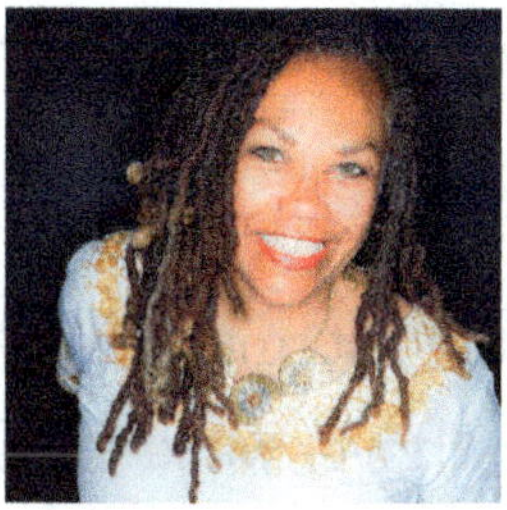

Terri is a 20+ year International Ghostwriter who has built a sizable portfolio of published books, blogs, articles, manuals, proposals, press releases and business correspondence. Her clients include motivational speakers such as world-renown Les Brown, high-profile public figures such as retired U.S. Senator Roland Burris and tons of ordinary people with extraordinary stories.

Terri's main writing interests are autobiographies and memoirs, health and wellness books, blogs and articles, and hosting therapeutic journaling retreats in the US and abroad.

Over the past decade, Terri's passion as a Health Advocate and End-Of-Life Strategist has guided many individuals to a healthier lifestyle. In 2000, she survived a heart attack at age 40 only to soon thereafter be diagnosed with a serious autoimmune disease called sarcoidosis. In 2012, she got rid of ALL her health issues by adopting a 100% raw, plant-based dietary lifestyle. To chronicle her journey to wellness, she wrote a book called, Get Your RAW On.

Currently, in her End-Of-Life Strategist role, Terri's mantra is "Helping baby-boomers thrive while alive, and leave a legacy, not a load, when time to go." She is developing a mobile app called 4th Quarter Living (4QL) to allow caregivers and the aging community in need of end-of-life services to connect with professionals who provide those products and services. Be it health & wellness, final expenses, final wishes, caregiving resources, estate planning, decluttering & downsizing, retirement income, and so much more, 4QL puts the information quickly and conveniently at one's fingertips, 24/7.

For more information on the development of the app, and the crowdfunding to bring it to the market, go to: https://TerriLiggins.com

# Resources by Terri Eileen Liggins

## Visit my website

https://TerriLiggins.com

The Law of Raw Institute for Balanced Healthy Living

4th Quarter Living

The Literary Front

Writing Out The Storm

## Follow me on social media

https://www.linkedin.com/in/writeful1/

https://www.facebook.com/LawOfRaw

https://www.facebook.com/TerriLigginsOfficial

https://www.instagram.com/terriliggins/

https://www.pinterest.com/teileenliggins

# Other books by Terri Eileen Liggins

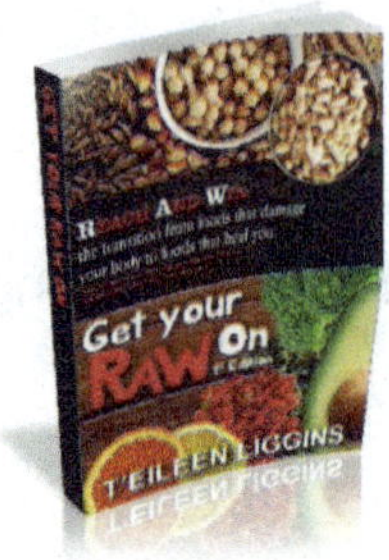

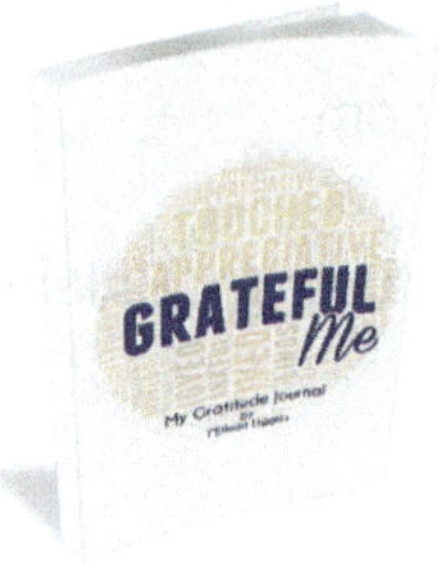

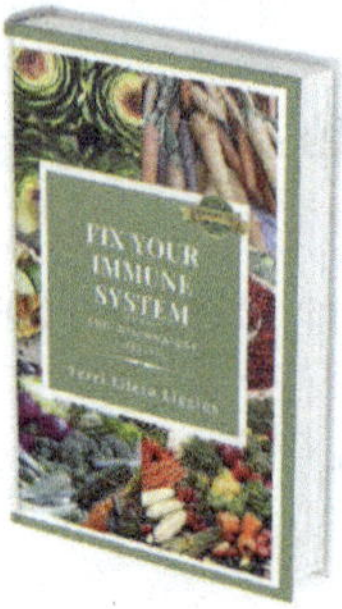


Coming Spring/Summer 2022…

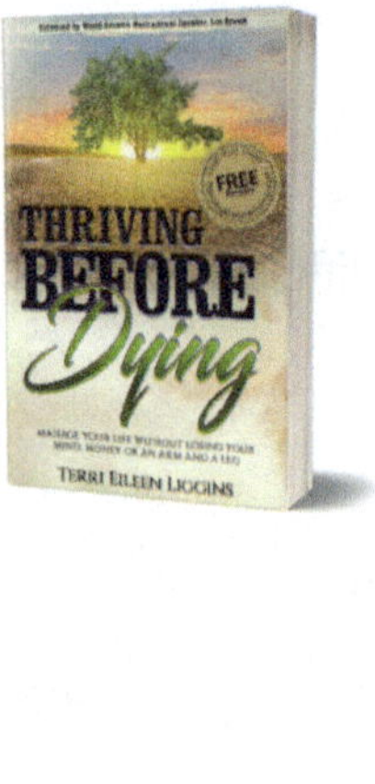

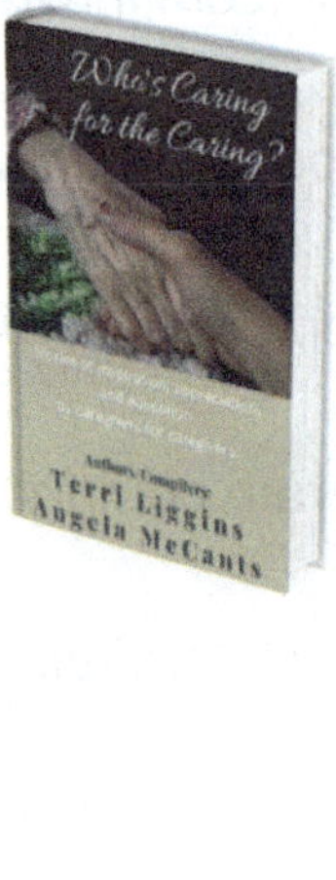

Made in the USA
Monee, IL
03 November 2026

67385888R00075